# JUICING FOR CANCER RECIPES BOOK

## *Delicious, Nutrient Rich Recipes for Fighting and Preventing Cancer*

## Dr. Stacy Holcolm

# Table of Contents

<u>**Chapter 5:**</u> Importance of supplements

<u>**Conclusion**</u>

# Introduction

Welcome to Juicing for Cancer Recipes, the ultimate guide to incorporating fresh and nutritious juices into your diet to help prevent and fight cancer. Juicing has long been known to be a powerful way to improve overall health and wellness, and can now be used as a part of an effective cancer prevention or treatment plan.

In this guide, we will provide you with recipes and tips specifically created to maximize the anti-cancer benefits of juicing. You will learn how to make delicious and nutrient-dense juices that can be tailored to your individual needs, as well as how to use juicing to support your body while undergoing cancer treatments. We will also discuss the importance of supplementation, and provide you with a list of supplements that can help you get the most out of your juicing.

Juicing is a simple and delicious way to add more nutritious fruits and vegetables to your diet, and can be beneficial for anyone looking to improve their overall health. Whether you are trying to prevent cancer or are currently undergoing treatment for cancer, incorporating fresh juices into your diet can have a powerful impact on your health. With this guide, you will have all the information you need to get started on a juicing plan that is tailored to your specific needs.

So let's get started! We hope you enjoy Juicing for Cancer Recipes and find the recipes and tips helpful in your journey to better health and wellness.

# Chapter 1

## The Benefits of Juicing for Cancer Patients

Here, we will be looking at the benefits of juicing for cancer patients and why it should be added to your recovery journey.

1. Juicing can provide numerous vitamins, minerals, and antioxidants that are not always available in other foods. This can be beneficial for cancer patients as these nutrients can help strengthen the immune system, reduce inflammation, and provide energy.

2. Juicing is an easy way to get a large amount of fruits and vegetables into one drink. This can provide a wide variety of

nutrients that can help cancer patients
stay strong and healthy.

3. Juicing can help cancer patients get
the necessary amount of vegetables and
fruits in their diet, even if they have
trouble chewing or swallowing solid food.

4. Juicing can help cancer patients
increase their intake of certain essential
nutrients, like lycopene and beta
carotene, which have been linked to a
reduced risk of certain types of cancer.

5. Juicing can help cancer patients
maintain their weight and keep their
bodies strong and healthy during
treatment.

6. Juicing can provide a delicious and
nutritious way to get the necessary
vitamins, minerals, and antioxidants
needed to help fight off cancer.

# Chapter 2

## Juicing Recipes for Cancer Patients

Here are some of the recipes for cancer patients and their methods of preparation.

**• Recipe 1: Carrot Beet Cleanser**
Ingredients:
• 2 large carrots
• 1 small beet
• 1/2 lemon
• 1/2 inch piece of fresh ginger
Instructions:
1. Wash and peel the carrots, beet, lemon, and ginger.
2. Cut the vegetables and fruit into small cubes.
3. Place the ingredients into a juicer and process until smooth.

4. Enjoy your Carrot Beet Cleanser!

## • Recipe 2: Green Detox Juice

Ingredients:
• 2 apples
• 2 cups spinach
• 1 cucumber
• 1/2 lemon
Instructions:
1. Wash and peel the apples, cucumber, and lemon.
2. Cut the vegetables and fruit into small cubes.
3. Place the ingredients into a juicer and process until smooth.
4. Enjoy your Green Detox Juice!

## • Recipe 3: Sweet Veggie Juice

Ingredients:
• 2 carrots
• 1/2 red bell pepper
• 1/2 beet
• 1/2 inch piece of fresh ginger

Instructions:
1. Wash and peel the carrots, bell pepper, beet, and ginger.
2. Cut the vegetables and fruit into small cubes.
3. Place the ingredients into a juicer and process until smooth.
4. Enjoy your Sweet Veggie Juice

## • Recipe 4: Kale and Carrot Juice

Ingredients
- 2 cups kale
- 2 carrots
- 2 apples
- 1/2 lemon
- 1/2 inch ginger root

Instructions
1. Wash and peel the carrots, apples, and ginger root.
2. Cut the apples, carrots, and ginger into small pieces.

3. Place all the ingredients into a blender or juicer.
4. Blend or juice the ingredients until smooth.
5. Serve and enjoy!

• **Recipe 5: Tomato and Celery Juice**
Ingredients:

-4 large tomatoes
-3 stalks of celery
-1/4 cup of fresh parsley
-1/2 lemon, juiced
-1/2 teaspoon of salt
-Freshly ground black pepper to taste

Instructions:

1. Wash tomatoes and celery and cut into pieces.

2. Place tomato and celery pieces into a juicer or blender.

3. Add parsley, lemon juice, salt, and pepper and blend until smooth.

4. Pour juice into a glass and serve. Enjoy!

**• Recipe 6: Ginger and Lemon Juice**
Ingredients:

-1 inch piece of fresh ginger, peeled and grated
-1 lemon, juiced
-1 tablespoon honey
-1 cup of water

Instructions:

1. In a small bowl, mix together the grated ginger and lemon juice.

2. Add the honey and stir until it is fully dissolved.

3. Pour in the water and mix until everything is combined.

4. Pour the mixture into a glass and enjoy.

## • **Recipe 7: Spinach and Pear Juice**

Ingredients:
-1 cup of fresh spinach
-2 pears, cored and diced
-1/2 cup of water
-1 teaspoon of honey (optional)

Instructions:
1. Rinse the spinach and place it in a blender.
2. Add the diced pears and water.
3. Blend the ingredients together until smooth.
4. Add honey if desired and blend again.

5. Strain the juice through a sieve or cheesecloth.
6. Serve the juice chilled and enjoy!

## • Recipe 8: Beet and Apple Juice

Ingredients:

- 2 medium beets, peeled and cut into cubes
- 2 apples, peeled and cut into cubes
- 1 cup of cold water
- 2 tablespoons of lemon juice (optional)

Instructions:

1. Place the beet cubes and apple cubes in a blender.

2. Add the cold water and lemon juice (if using).

3. Blend until smooth.

4. Strain the juice through a fine mesh sieve into a bowl or pitcher.

5. Serve the juice chilled or over ice. Enjoy!

# Chapter 3

## Tips for Juicing with Cancer

1. Talk to your healthcare provider before starting a juicing routine.
2. Choose organic produce when possible to limit exposure to pesticides.
3. Use a variety of fruits and vegetables in your juice.
4. Avoid juices high in sugar.
5. Drink your juice right away as it loses nutrients over time.
6. Consider adding herbs and spices to your juice, such as ginger or turmeric, to boost the health benefits.
7. Incorporate cruciferous vegetables such as kale, cabbage, and broccoli into your juices.
8. If you're on chemotherapy, avoid consuming juices with high amounts of

vitamin K, such as kale, as it can interfere with the effectiveness of the treatment.

9. Be sure to include some healthy fats in your juice, such as flaxseed, chia seeds or coconut oil.

10. Start with small amounts of juice and gradually increase the amount over time to avoid digestive upset.

# Chapter 4

## Supplements for juicing

1. Wheatgrass: Wheatgrass is high in chlorophyll and is believed to be a powerful antioxidant that helps to detoxify the body and fight off cancer cells.

2. Dandelion Greens: Dandelion greens are packed with antioxidants and have anti-cancer properties that help to fight off cancer cells and reduce the risk of tumor growth.

3. Kale: Kale is rich in vitamin A, vitamin C, and other cancer-fighting antioxidants that help to boost the body's immunity and fight off cancer cells.

4. Spinach: Spinach is another nutrient-dense leafy green that contains powerful antioxidants that help to reduce the risk of cancer.

5. Beetroot: Beetroot is high in antioxidants and has anti-cancer properties that help to reduce the risk of cancer and protect the body from the damaging effects of free radicals.

6. Carrots: Carrots are high in beta-carotene and other cancer-fighting antioxidants that help to fight off cancer cells and reduce the risk of tumor growth.

7. Garlic: Garlic has anti-cancer properties that help to fight off cancer cells and boost the body's immunity.

8. Ginger: Ginger has anti-inflammatory properties that help to reduce the risk of

cancer and protect the body from the damaging effects of free radicals.

# Chapter 5

## Importance of Supplements

Supplements are an important part of juicing with cancer recipes, as they can help to provide additional nutrients and antioxidants that may help to support overall health and wellbeing. Supplements can provide additional vitamins and minerals that may not be found in fresh produce, as well as additional antioxidants that could help to fight the negative effects of cancer. Additionally, supplements can help to boost the immune system, which is especially important for those fighting cancer. Supplements can also provide additional energy and help to reduce inflammation, both of which are important for anyone fighting cancer.

Finally, supplements can help to provide essential fatty acids that may be lacking in the diet, which can help to improve overall health.

## Conclusion

In conclusion, the Juicing for Cancer Recipes Book is a great resource for anyone looking to make healthy, nutritious meals that can help fight cancer. It is full of delicious recipes and helpful information, and it is a great way to get started with juicing. The book includes a variety of recipes that are easy to follow and can be tailored to fit individual needs. The book also offers helpful advice on selecting and storing produce, and how to get the most out of each juice. Furthermore, the book provides information on the benefits of juicing and how it can help to promote health and wellbeing. Juicing for Cancer Recipes Book is an excellent resource for anyone looking to make healthier, cancer fighting meals.